teaching
people,
not
poses

12 principles for teaching
yoga with integrity

jay fields

jay fields

Cover design by Bernadette Galione

Author photo by Debbie Baxter

For all my teachers and students.

jay fields

12 Principles

1. Be yourself.
2. Practice.
3. Show your vulnerability and your expertise.
4. Teach from your own experience.
5. If you don't know, say you don't know.
6. Stay in your body.
7. Don't take it all so seriously.
8. Remember that your students are people.
9. Learn anatomy.
10. Plan enough so that you can be spontaneous.
11. Remember who and what supports you.
12. Don't try to please everyone.

Introduction

As for many people, my yoga teacher training changed my life. I came alive to parts of myself that had never before been fostered, and I learned a tremendous amount about teaching yoga postures and philosophy.

I did not, however, learn how to *teach people*—how to accommodate a room full of people with distinct abilities, personalities, needs and preferences. Or how to teach a pose as a means of connecting on deeper levels to the wholeness of one's experience, rather than as an end in itself.

Nor did I learn how to make space for my own humanity within my role as a yoga teacher—how to attend to all of my own insecurities, blind spots, fears and desires. How to get out of my own way enough to teach a class, and how to show up to a room full of people on the days when I didn't even want to get out of bed.

This skill of learning how to convey information about the vast practice of yoga as one human being to other human beings came over many years of trial by fire in the studio, and just as many years of self-study, regular yoga practice and life experience.

One could argue that this kind of learning can only happen in this way—experientially. You've got to give yourself years to let this being a teacher thing get into your bones. And yet, though no one can walk the road of teaching for you, I can put up some signposts for things to look out for along the way.

The 12 principles are meant to be that: guides for how to approach your teaching as a practice in itself. Because if you're truly engaged in the process of teaching, both your teaching and your self will continually evolve and change over time. And not change as in "get better," but change as in *become more you.*

The following pages are meant to offer you a foundation for becoming the fullest expression of yourself as a teacher in the studio and as yourself in your life.

I invite you to consider the questions posed with each principle, to try the principles out in the studio and to use them to help direct you to your own true offering as a remarkable yoga teacher.

It's my belief that the more yoga teachers who endeavor to show up to their teaching with as much integrity as they can, the more the yoga community is served, and the yoga lineage honored.

May this book inspire you and all you teach!

1. Be yourself.

When I first started doing yoga I thought it would make me a better person. In fact, in the first year that I practiced, I would say my life felt brighter and more manageable than ever before. I was dropping the edge of competition I had grown up with as a gymnast, I was learning how to be gentler with myself and I was feeling more positive and engaged with the world in general.

If *taking* yoga could do this, what could *teaching* yoga do?

This wasn't necessarily a conscious thought, but I sought out teaching because somewhere in me I thought it was the sure path to enlightenment in this life. Well, maybe not enlightenment, but at least a life that wasn't so freaking messy and uncomfortable.

Little did I know at that point that yoga isn't about making your life more *manageable*. In fact, within a few months of taking my teacher training I was divorced and totally at a loss for what to do with my life. How's that for not messy?

But I had an idea of what a yoga teacher should be like, and I went through that time in my life playing the role of yoga teacher. I focused on the positive, told myself the heartbreak would only make me stronger and that everything would be ok again some day (i.e. easy, comfortable and manageable). To put it succinctly, I spiritually bypassed the emotional shit storm that was raging under the surface. I'd walk into my class as if my whole world wasn't falling to pieces, and I would teach poses. God only knows what I said during those classes, but I'm sure it sounded like total bull.

In the fourteen years I've been teaching, I've been through more break ups than I'd like to think about, more moves than I can count, chronic illness for a few years, deaths of loved ones, a miscarriage and a roll over car accident. I've also fallen in love more than once, earned a graduate degree, studied with inspiring teachers, found a rich and trustworthy relationship with my inner guidance, and experienced many deeply, profoundly loving moments.

In short, I've been a human being.

In looking back from this vantage point, it turns out that my yoga practice as a student and as a teacher hasn't made me more enlightened, it's simply made me more *myself*. And lo and behold, my self isn't as one-dimensional and together as my vision of the perfect yoga teacher.

Thank god.

Because I've come to understand that the very things I used to try to hide are what make me more interesting, and also what enable me to connect with other people in a way that is real and meaningful. I've discovered that the only person who thinks I should have my shit together when I walk into a room full of people is me. And I've come to accept that being myself, even if I'm sometimes needy or jerky or scared or sad, is far more preferable (and less exhausting) than constantly trying to outrun myself.

And that feels good. Mostly. It also feels vulnerable. To stand up in front of a group of people week after week as *me* still scares me. It's funny, until a year ago I've always been looking for a real job, something I could call my career. Not because I don't think teaching yoga is a credible career, but because I think teaching yoga is flipping scary. I wanted to believe that I could find something that I love to do as much as I love teaching, but that isn't so confronting of all the tender places in my heart and spirit. (And that also pays better!)

But through this ever-evolving journey to myself that has been yoga, I've found that this kind of confrontation with the grace and grit of life is exactly *why* I love teaching yoga, and I wouldn't have it any other way. And it's not that I think that teaching poses isn't important—I love *asana* and am a total geek about anatomy—it's just that I've become more interested in how teaching and practicing yoga offers such a tremendous opportunity to bump up against my deeper self in ways that aren't always comfortable but are often liberating.

So you know how your students get cranky when you can't teach and there's a sub there? That's because there's something about *you* that they love and respond to. Anyone can teach a series of poses, but only you can be you. Trust that. Trust that your students are attracted to your classes because of who you are, and bring more of yourself to your teaching.

But don't do it for your students, do it for you so that you can have more of yourself in everything you do. Even if you're not the self you thought you'd grow up to be.

Going Deeper

To be honest, I'm still trying to figure this whole "be yourself" thing out. In part because I'm continually learning just who my self is. In part because I'm still working on getting out of my own way enough so that I can just be that self. Seems like it should be so basic and simple, and yet it's ridiculously hard to do.

There are different levels to this conversation about how to be yourself when you're teaching. The deeper level is about doing the emotional processing and personal work needed to dismiss the ways you resist your true self being seen. This level is best addressed experientially through counseling, individual mentoring and workshops. You can't just write or talk about this level, you have to participate.

The more superficial level of being yourself, which can be addressed in writing, is about not being afraid to show your personality when you teach. It's about being *you* rather than playing the role of yoga teacher.

As I said before, I've definitely played the role. It's hard not to start out there as you begin to find yourself in your teaching. But ask yourself, do you have a teacher persona and an everyday persona that are quite different? If so, why?

So here are just three things that come up for me when thinking about ways that you can be yourself as you teach. They're simple, but they go a long way in setting the stage for the deeper work of being your self:

1. Dress the way you want to dress.

It seems almost laughable to have to say this, but with the commoditization of yoga and branded booties everywhere, it's important to remember that you don't have to buy into it all. Unless, of course, it's authentically your style. Granted, you're a professional, so I wouldn't recommend risqué tops and super short shorts. Nor would I recommend the sweat pants you wear around the house that have stains and holes all over them, but don't feel like your students expect you to look a certain way. Well, maybe they do, but who cares?

If your shirt doesn't have a yoga brand name on it, great. If you've had those pants for 17 years and you love them, great. Want to wear a dress over pants? Great. As long as you can move in them and they're not revealing, wear whatever clothes you want.

When you dress the way you want to dress, you're not only showing more of you, but you're also showing your students that they don't have to buy into the branding of yoga either. It's a subtle, yet strong way to demonstrate that yoga isn't about having the perfect tank top or the perfect pose, but about letting your clothes and your poses be an expression of who you are.

2. Don't' be afraid to mix in some profane with the sacred.

I don't mean cause a scene or be an inappropriate asshole, again, I just mean be your self. Off the mat, I am silly and sarcastic, and I'm known to have a bit of a potty mouth, so in my classes I sometimes do a ridiculous little leprechaun dance when I'm excited, I make up stupid names for poses or sequences, and I occasionally drop a four-letter word when making a point (such as my favorite instruction from Erich Schiffmann to totally fuck up your pose so that you can find it again as your own).

That said, recognize that there's a fine line between seeking attention for yourself and bringing to your students' attention that you (and thus they) have permission to be yourself, as dorky, profane or generally "non-yogic" as that may be.

3. Use your voice.

I don't mean finding your empowered and authentic voice (though yes, do this!). I simply mean use *your* voice. Like the one you use when you talk to your friends, not some sing-songy or stylized voice of a yoga teacher.

I remember years ago going to a *vinyasa* class where the teacher said "downward facing dog" as if she were a cheesy sportscaster on the evening news...(deepened voice) downward (pause and then higher tone) facing (deepening her voice again) dog. Do you know how many times a teacher says downward facing dog in the course of a *vinyasa* class? Even though the sequence was brilliant, I nearly had to leave because the cheese factor of her tone was driving me crazy.

Believe me, *your* voice is what your students will enjoy listening to the most, and is how you can best convey whatever it is you want to share.

What parts of your personality do you already convey well through your teaching?

In what ways might you compromise yourself to fit a role or to please others?

What one thing could you do differently to have more of yourself while you teach?

2. Practice.

You gotta' practice. Period.

That's kinda' it.

But I'll expound a bit.

I remember a few years ago going to a class with a teacher I had never met. When we were talking before class I commented on how it's nice sometimes to go to a class and to have someone else hold space for you. He agreed, and added that he could count on one hand the number of times he had practiced at home on his own. In that moment I knew I would never go to his class again. I even considered walking out right then and there.

You might think that was a jerky judgment to make, but I don't. Why would I practice with someone who has no practice of his own? That would be like having an actor who plays a doctor on TV prescribe a course of treatment for me; he knows the words from a script he's read, but he really has no idea what he's talking about from his own depth of knowledge or experience.

I want to be upfront: I'm not perfect about practicing everyday. I go through funks when I don't practice for a couple of days at a time. And there were times early in my teaching, particularly the year after my divorce, when the last thing I wanted was to be on my mat in my own company with no one else around. I would go weeks and weeks without practicing then.

I will also be the first person to admit that these times when I don't practice are not my best days—as a person or as a teacher. These are days that I am either uncomfortable in or disconnected from my body. I'm usually avoiding having a specific feeling. Scratch that. I'm *always* avoiding having a specific feeling. Avoiding an uncomfortable feeling is really the only reason I don't practice.

Whether it's sadness or anger or fear or judgment or just that general anxiety that if I take the time to practice that I won't be able to get to all the important stuff on my to do list for the day—I don't practice because I'm avoiding myself, not the actual poses.

By the way, that last excuse is one of the biggest loads of bull I continually try to feed myself. Really? What on my to do list is possibly more important than taking the time to anchor myself in my own presence? Without that presence, I'm really not actually living my life, no matter how much I get done. Instead I'm being run by thoughts, patterns and habituated ways of being. And without a felt connection to myself, I can't truly connect to or be present with anyone else. This is an obstacle for teaching, not to mention for genuine relating of any sort.

That's not to say that if I practice in the morning I remain a beacon of presence for the entirety of the day. Hardly. But it does deepen the rut of knowing how to get my mind to shut up, which is a good rut to deepen. And it does give me more conscious awareness of what's happening emotionally and energetically behind the thoughts that I'm thinking, which helps me to feel more grounded (even if it's grounded in a funk). It also helps me to actually *feel* my body, which is imperative in terms of being in touch with what I need—and with what my students need.

I've discovered in the last year in particular that I'm far less tolerant of the emotional shut down, the energetic dullness and the physical tightness I feel from not practicing than I am of all the potentially uncomfortable feelings I could meet by going to my mat. I consider this a turning point, and I have noticed a difference in my teaching; even if I can only take 15 minutes on my mat in the morning, I feel I have more integrity to offer because of it.

And this is what practicing is all about: integrity. Your integrity as a person and as a teacher, and the integrity that your teaching has to offer the yoga community. Without going to your mat day after day, you can't know the poses from the inside out. More importantly, you can't possibly know yourself from the inside out. And if you don't know the poses or your self in this way, how can you even begin to share the poses with others, or know others in the poses?

Practice is not about being perfect. It's about being yourself. It's about getting past your lines of defense to find the soft, chewy, sweet center. It's about being able to be with yourself when you're in the pits and when you're off the wall giddy. It's about growing your sensitivity for what it feels like to be in your body. It's about noticing what you do to try to escape, and what works to settle in. It's about gaining a broad spectrum of experience as a human being in a body, so you can connect more with other human beings in their full experience of themselves in a body.

Going Deeper

I think one of the hardest things for me as a teacher to remember about my personal yoga practice is that it's just that: personal.

Right now it's two hours until I teach my class and I haven't practiced yet this morning. I can feel how I want to go to my mat so that I can get centered for the sake of my students and to figure out some sort of sequence, as opposed to just using the time to get what I need for myself and trusting that me simply being present will inform the best possible class.

So let's start there: your practice is not for your teaching. It's for *you*. It's not for fixing yourself or figuring out how to be a better teacher or even for accomplishing a certain pose. It's for being *you*.

All the other stuff like being a more-informed teacher and becoming more adept at handstand will just happen if you practice. Becoming yourself through your practice, though, takes creating intentional space for yourself.

That said, one of the biggest obstacles to practicing at home is feeling like it has to look a certain way; you get centered and peaceful and then perform a warm-up, a series of standing poses, some seated poses and twists, *pranayama*, meditation…you know, well-rounded.

Some days that is great—as a teacher it's good to have a well-rounded practice and to really be familiar with the poses. And yet, if the intention is to practice being a present human being, the practice doesn't always look like "yoga."

Some days my practice looks like taking a cup of tea to my mat and sipping while I read poetry. Some days it looks like curling up under my yoga blanket and crying and snotting all over my mat. Some days it looks like cranking tunes and going back and forth between poses and booty shaking. And some days it looks like a very purposeful sequence of dialed-in postures followed by a long meditation.

The thing is, there can be just as much unconsciousness in practicing the same way every morning as there can be in not practicing at all. It's so easy to come to your mat and to just go through the motions without ever truly feeling the fullness of the present moment.

Why do you practice?

How can you tell the difference between when you're practicing for yourself and when you're practicing for the sake of your students?

What is one rule you have for yourself around practicing? Break it!

3. Show your vulnerability and your expertise.

The other day I walked into class and started as I always do—checking in with folks and asking them what they needed. The unanimous vote was neck and shoulders.

"Oh good," I thought to myself. "That's exactly what I need."

My left rhomboid was doing its thing again—the thing it does when it seizes up and renders it nearly impossible for me to turn my head and just plain uncomfortable to be in my body. I call it my heartstring—it gets all knotted up when I'm really scared or sad about something.

Through the years I have learned some incredible techniques for getting a direct stretch to this area through yoga, so I felt confident as I began class with a series from my collection of upper back and neck stretches.

About a half hour in to the systematic unwinding of this area, I noticed that my heartstring was still just as tightly knotted as ever. The truth is, though I've learned a bunch of ways to stretch and strengthen this area over the years, I've also learned that no amount of stretching or strengthening makes this pain go away when I experience it in this way. The only thing that makes this particular pain go away is for me to crawl into bed and have a big, snotty cry and a deep, drooly nap.

So as we came back into *tadasana* to check in with how we were feeling, I shared this with my students—how sometimes a good cry is a better release than any yoga stretch can ever be. And that going home to have a big cry was exactly what I intended to do because I was really scared about something that was happening in my life.

After class one of the women who had been to my class for the first time that night came up to me and introduced herself as a fellow yoga teacher. Instead of commenting on the wonderfully geeky poses we did to get straight at the spots in her shoulder she had asked for, what she said instead was, "I was so surprised that you said what you did about needing a big cry—and I loved it. I thought, wow, she just said the one thing that we all do but no one wants to admit to. What a beautiful gift you gave us."

Your students go to a yoga class because everyone has knots and tight spots they need to work out, and they want someone who is expert enough to help them to do that. But the truth is, your students also go to a yoga class because they want to feel a *connection*. Whether it's through moving and breathing in your body or through the softening that comes through being reflected to yourself by another person's words or actions, we all want to feel like we're not alone.

No amount of technical expertise can create that connection. Connection requires vulnerability.

If I had wanted to remain "the expert," I could have said some smart comment about how we all hold emotions in our bodies and how it's ok to cry and let them out. My inner tough girl would have preferred me do this. Speaking in this way keeps me safely hidden and distant. But that's all a comment like that does—hides me and creates distance between my students and I. It lets me pretend that I'm more evolved than I am, and conveys to my students that if they just practiced enough they, too, would not have to ever feel scared or sad again. And that's just a load of shit.

So the seeming paradox is that being a human being and showing vulnerability actually *adds* to expertise. Mind you, I'm not asking them to hold me while I cry. I'm not processing my stuff with them in the studio. I'm not telling them the story behind why I'm scared. I'm just being candid that I'm scared as hell and I need to go home and hug my pillow.

In so doing I acknowledge the part of them who has felt the same way—maybe even in that very moment—and give them permission to be more of themselves on and off their mat. All of this vulnerability is presented within a killer *asana* sequence with spot-on adjustments to show them that I might be scared, but I still know what I'm doing.

And isn't that kind of true for most of us? Just because you have a tender heart doesn't mean you don't also have sharp skills.

And so, vulnerability without skill is just as useless as skill without vulnerability. Both need to be present to be a truly remarkable teacher of people, not poses.

Going Deeper

I don't know about you, but the people I respect the most are the people who I think are absolute experts at what they do, *and* who show their vulnerability.

Brene' Brown is a brilliant social scientist who studies shame, but I love her work so much because of how she reveals her own insecurities and idiosyncracies along with her research.

Danielle LaPorte has the most grounded, get real advice when it comes to being a spitfire in business, and she puts herself out there in a big, personal and unapologetic way.

Melanie Murphy on the eighth season of the television show *So You Think You Can Dance* blew me away as one of the most gifted dancers I've ever seen. Yes, she has impeccable technical expertise as a dancer, but it was the way that she exposed her heart and soul as she danced that made America vote her the best dancer that season.

Through being vulnerably themselves in their own way, these women give me permission to be myself, which is a gift in itself. But then they also have the ability to shine forth their excellence and offer tips or inspiration for just how I can be more excellent at what I do, too. This combo of vulnerability and expertise is all about creating meaningful connection and cultivating street cred, not just about being an expert on paper.

So how do you find your expertise and vulnerability as a yoga teacher? Well, your expertise comes through what you learn in your practice. Not just your *asana* practice on the mat, but your meditation practice and any other practices you engage in that are about self-awareness and growth.

Your vulnerability then comes from revealing who you really are from what you've discover about yourself through your practices and through the present moment of your teaching.

So much of how to be a teacher who has integrity is simply about how to find this balance of vulnerability and expertise. In terms of putting it into practice, look to some of the other principles for how to *Teach People, Not Poses:* speak from your own experience, stay in your body, drop your plan and be spontaneous, don't try to please everyone. All of these things require vulnerability and also have the potential to showcase expertise.

Just so you know, it's going to feel uncomfortable and scary. That's why it's called vulnerability. And if you're anything like me, your inner tough girl or boy is going to want nothing to do with it. But trying to hide your vulnerability doesn't really work—it always shows regardless of whether you admit it or not, and if you don't own it, your vulnerability can be interpreted in a way that you don't intend (as arrogance, ignorance, jerkiness, or flakiness).

If you don't allow for your vulnerability then it means you have a shield up. And if you have a shield up, it means you can't really create true connection between you and your students. And this connection, along with trust and acceptance, is what people want more than any expertly crafted sequence of poses.

Trust that. And trust your own vulnerability to be what infuses your expert teaching with humanity and heart in a way that is greatly needed.

From the list of principles, which one feels the most vulnerable to you? Which one makes you want to hide? Or throw up? Or both?

Give yourself permission to start to flirt with your vulnerability: Class full of new students? Tell them you're feeling shy and nervous. That one student who just wants a work out and who sits right in front of you to intimidate you is in class today? Read the poem anyway. Didn't have time to plan a class? Don't fall back on what you taught the day before—feel into what's in the present moment and let it guide you.

4. Teach from your own experience.

The natural consequence of being yourself, practicing, and being willing to show your expertise and your vulnerability is being able to teach from your own experience. This could mean a few different things, but the gist is this: Don't teach anything in your class that you don't know in your body.

Having said that, let me break this down a bit more, as there are a few different aspects of speaking from your own experience as a yoga teacher.

First, there's your experience of the poses themselves. The best teachers don't use the same textbook cues for the same poses over and over. Assuming you're practicing, your embodied understanding of the poses always evolves, and your cues become more nuanced, interesting and *useful*.

Instead of "lift your leg," you can say, "Feel how when you lift your leg more from your inner thigh you can keep your hips level and extend longer through to your heel." You can say it this way because you've felt it in your own body.

Your experience of the poses from your own practice allows you to speak to all the ways your students will want to "cheat" in the pose to avoid sensation, as well as all the possibilities for opening and strengthening and the million other things that happen in any given shape. This ability to speak to a wide range of experiences from your own experience helps you to teach and to *connect to* a room full of people with different bodies and different experiences.

Then there's the more vulnerable side of things—speaking from your experience as a human being. I want to be clear that I don't mean "talking about yourself." What I'm talking about here is the difference between talking *about* yourself, which is telling stories about yourself in a way that often doesn't serve anyone (including yourself), and speaking *from* your experience, which means letting your experience of being a human being inform how you convey information in a way that serves the people listening (and usually yourself).

For example, when I do reversed triangle pose I get agitated and super judgmental of myself because it's a really hard pose for me. Rather than tell my students this (which, depending on the situation, I sometimes will), I can use that experience to inform what I say to them while they're holding the pose: "Notice if you're getting agitated. Watch if your mind turns to judgments."

By saying those comments I'm not implying that I think everyone has the same experience in the pose that I do, but I think it's pretty safe to assume I'm not the only one who has that experience. Either way, offering something from my own experience invites my students to discover for themselves what they feel in the pose. This makes the practice more grounded and connected to what's real for the students rather than a game of adult Simon Says where everyone moves in the same way without feeling what's really going on.

Lastly, there's speaking from your own experience of the present moment. This is tapping into what you notice goes on for you as you teach, what you see in your students as they practice, and what's happening in the collective field. This is when you say, "Relax your jaw" every time you notice yourself gripping your own jaw. This is when you say, "Make sure you're breathing" when you can see, hear and feel that people in the room are holding their breath. This is when you use the car alarm that suddenly starts blaring during *savasana* to speak to how to stay present with yourself when the world is inherently full of distractions and annoyances.

This is one of my favorite parts of teaching. It makes teaching feel like improvisational art. It's terrifying and so very alive to teach from your experience of the present moment. In this place planning becomes obsolete at best, a roadblock at worst. You have the opportunity to experience deep connection with self, other and Mystery.

This is what I aspire to on my best days. It's what makes for the classes when more than one student comes up at the end and says, "It feels like you taught that class just for me."

That's the beautiful paradox of speaking from your own experience—the more you source your teaching from your personal experience, the more personal it becomes for everyone else.

Going Deeper

When I was writing my graduate thesis, I had a major case of writer's block. I had no idea how to write about concepts associated with spiritual enlightenment without sounding like a total jackass or overtly contradicting things that I had written about other spiritual concepts. Spiritual "truths" are like that—tricky and contradictory.

I took a break from writing and had tea with a friend of mine who is a Buddhist monk. He set me straight. "Jay," he explained, "when writing about spiritual concepts, you've got to be candid about what level of experience you're talking about them from. If you're not enlightened and your talking about enlightenment, you've got to tell your reader that this is your current understanding of something you have not yet experienced."

And with that, my writer's block dissolved. All I had to do was be clear that I (big shock) was indeed not enlightened and that I was writing about my understanding of enlightenment from my place left of there on the spectrum of spiritual understanding.

This, I think, is a useful thing to apply to the metaphysical and spiritual side of teaching yoga. Nothing makes me more annoyed than to have a yoga teacher spew spiritual truths as if she has personally lived them. Unless she has. And then I consider it a true gift that she can articulate that and an honor to be able to learn with her.

Many of us got in to teaching yoga because we are aware that the practice offers more than just physical benefits, but teaching about the spiritual, emotional and mental benefits is one of the most challenging things to do. It's a fine line between being inspiring and being fake. That line is made up of your own experience and your ability to speak from it.

The thing is, your students can sense when you're regurgitating something you read or are just channeling a spiritual teacher's words. And if your students are anything like me, it kind of makes them want to throw up.

I'm not saying don't share readings and beautiful quotes from other people, but do ground them in your own experience. What do they bring up for you? How does it make you feel? Why did you share that today? Where do you see that play out in your life or in the studio? This is where being willing to show your vulnerability comes in handy.

Whether teaching the physical, spiritual, mental or emotional aspect of yoga I find that the same formula applies:

1. Notice what you are experiencing.

2. Assume you're not the only one.

3. Share it in a way that might inspire someone else to notice what he is experiencing.

You can apply this to the way a sequence feels in your body (even if you've commandeered the sequence from another teacher's class), the emotion a reading brings up for you, a thought you have as you watch a student attempt a challenging pose...*any* type of experience, as long as it's yours.

For example, a teacher friend of mine told me last night after her candlelit *yin* class that I attended that she normally has music on and teaching without it kind of made her feel exposed. I told her that I bet she wasn't the only one in the room who felt that way because of the silence, and suggested that it would have been an interesting thing to comment on. "Notice if not having any music in the background tonight makes you feel more at ease or more exposed."

Not everyone would have shared her experience, but in my friend sharing from her own sense of exposure she would have invited her students to be curious about what was happening for them. And that's kind of what yoga is all about—present moment awareness and authentic acknowledgement of where you are on all spectrums so that you can make real connections with yourself and with others.

That means as a teacher you need to be as curious as you can about your own experience, as honest as you can about your own understanding of what's real for you and as articulate as you can be in conveying it so as to create a point of connection with your students.

With that, an extra word of advice—don't feel like you have to juggle all the different layers of an experience at once. There's a lot going on in any given moment. It can be hard, especially as a new teacher, to track yourself on more than one experiential level at once. Just pick the one that's most available and most interesting to you and start there.

Over time you'll find that you can articulate your experience on different levels more fluidly. As your experience and your understanding of your experience evolves, so too will your teaching.

Get in touch with your own experience in this moment. How do you feel? What are you thinking about?

Assuming you're not the only one who's ever had this experience, how would you articulate this as you teach in a way that might help your students become more self-aware?

What asana might either metaphorically represent or evoke this feeling?

5. If you don't know, say you don't know.

A number of years ago I went to see Buddhist teacher Noah Levine read from his book *Dharma Punx* at Powell's Bookstore in Portland, Oregon. I was so impressed by his presence, by his wisdom at such a young age, and by just how edgy and real he was.

When he opened the floor for questions after his reading, people raised their hands and he offered thoughtful responses to their questions. Then one guy toward the back raised his hand and asked a question—I don't even remember the question itself, I just remember that it was epic. It was one of those questions that is part personal story, part showing off how much you already know about the topic you're asking about and then part stick it to you in the what-are-you-gonna'-say-to-*that* kind of way.

I remember expectantly turning my head back to Noah, shrinking a bit for his sake, and thinking, "God, I'm so glad someone didn't ask me that question because I would have no idea what to say."

Noah pondered it earnestly for a few moments, and then said, "Huh. I have no idea."

I instantly liked him even more. His credibility went way up in my book.

In truth, it was a huge turning point for me. (Obviously, if I still remember it so vividly years later!) "Wow," I thought. "If I think more highly of Noah for saying that he doesn't know, maybe I could do that rather than trying to come up with some partial answer at best, and wrong answer at worst when I'm put on the spot in that way."

I don't think I'm alone in disliking not knowing something. For me it's in part because I like to fancy myself a bit of a smarty—and I like to fancy myself a bit of a smarty because I told myself a long time ago that people will like me better if I'm smart. So it used to be a huge edge for me to not know the answer to something because I was scared that it would mean that I would disappoint that person and they wouldn't like me.

I actually remember as a kid making up directions to someplace for some stranger who stopped me on the street because I thought I "should" know. Yeah, like that made me look smart when the guy ended up more lost! And like my "directions" actually helped that poor man out in any way. Seeing Noah that night and finding that I respected him more for his honesty helped shift my desire to always have an answer.

The other part of it, though, is that I think people collectively just really hate uncertainty. We'd like to think that *someone* has the answer. This certainly goes for the Big Questions in Life, but just in general, too.

I'm thinking of a student who recently asked me what I thought is causing the chronic pain in her shoulder. Behind her question I felt some anxiety that it's something that will limit her range of motion or cause pain for a long time, or fear that she's doing something to damage the joint. Consciously or not, I felt like she wanted me to take away her uncertainty so she wouldn't have to feel anxiety or fear, or so that she could "do" something about it. A recovering people-pleaser, I really wanted to help her by having an answer that would make it better.

Plus, my own insecurities came up. For a moment the thought, "What kind of yoga teacher am I if I can't say what's causing that?" Well, a limited one. I might have an undergraduate degree in Kinesiology (the study of human movement), and over a dozen years of yoga practice and teaching, but I'm not a doctor. Trying to help either one of us out of the discomfort of our uncertainty by coming up with an answer for the sake of an answer could actually cause her more damage and suffering.

This is particularly risky when it comes to questions about injuries, but coming up with an answer just to have an answer for *any* type of question—the meaning of a *sutra*, the way to build flexibility in a specific muscle, or the best book to read about meditation—is simply not helpful.

The gist: have the courage and humility to say you don't know!

And then you can follow that up a few different ways:

1. Ask them what they think. This is what Noah did with epic-question-guy, and I thought it was brilliant. This is good for when it's clear that the person is seeking your opinion about something that it might be more helpful for them to consider what they actually think or feel about it.

2. Tell them you'll find out and get back to them. It might be something that you know you have written down somewhere or that you know just the person who would have the answer. This shows that you might not be able to answer them in the moment, but that you are interested in knowing the answer and in helping them out.

3. Suggest they ask someone else and then come back to you with what they learned. This is good for the questions about injuries. Tell them to make an appointment with their doctor and report back. Again, you can be humble and ready to learn more, and willing to work collaboratively with your student in uncertainty.

Going Deeper

If you've played at all with not planning your classes, or you've spilled your tea on your carefully crafted lesson plan in the middle of teaching, then you've experienced that dreadful moment when you suddenly have absolutely no freaking clue what to do next.

You look at the clock—46 more minutes? Shit! You hope your panic and shortened breaths don't show as your students are sweating it out in an extra long down dog while you desperately try to figure something out.

Not knowing is so scary! And it's also super cool because it means you're not limiting your options by thinking you have the answer. Because if you're honest with yourself and trying to live your life as fully as you can, the reality is that you're going to be in this place of not knowing a whole hell of a lot. So you might as well make friends with it.

The first thing to do is realize that any time you don't know the answer to something, it's a good time to check in with your guidance or intuition. Rather than frantically going through past lesson plans in your head or racking your brain for what your teacher would do in this situation, get in touch with your body in the present moment and ask, "What's next?"

Usually you will find that your body, through its felt sense and mirror neurons, knows what it wants to feel next. "Oh, time for a hamstring stretch." And then you might imagine or feel your body doing a certain pose. Trust that this will feel good to your students, too, and go there.

Sometimes the signal for guidance is fuzzy and it doesn't come through. In my experience, this is when panic steps it up a notch. I've definitely found myself standing in front of my class, eyes closed, asking guidance what to do next only to get no perceptible answer.

And yes, I do actually stand in front of my class with them standing in front of me in *tadasana* and take a few moments to close my eyes and to not say anything while I discern what's next. It's a good teaching moment for what it looks like to get more comfortable with being willing to not know, and for going inward for answers.

In cases like this sometimes I'll open my eyes and say, "Hell, I don't know what's next! But you do." I'll remind my students to ask their body and not their head, and then to just do whatever they feel is next without thinking about it too much. This is a great way for people to see how much they actually *do* know what's next, or how they know what they want but second guess it, or how they know but choose something else because it will look better or because that's what someone else is doing.

I do this a lot in my class, and not just when I don't know what's next, but because I really want to support my students in finding *their* practice rather than just robotically responding to someone else's cues. I'll sometimes offer some possibilities, and sometimes not. I'll also offer that an option is to simply stand there and not know what's next—since I've done this many times in front of them, they know I mean it when I give them permission. And hell, that standing there not knowing is in its own way just as juicy and useful as any pose.

Remember, your job isn't to make your students more comfortable in every way or to hold their hand through the whole practice, your job is to be yourself and to support your students in being themselves.

What do you do when you're in a moment of not knowing while you teach?

What do you do when you see a student seeming confused about something?

How can you make more space for not knowing in your classes?

6. Stay in your body.

It seems like an odd thing to have to say that staying in your body is one of the principles—as if aliens or some strange force were ever-present and threatening to whisk you out of your body. But in a way it's true. It's just that it's not aliens or a strange force; it's your own mind.

I can't even begin to tell you how much I hang out in my head. I like to try to figure things out, manage, plot, scheme, control, arrange, strategize, manipulate, direct, engineer, plan...

My students always comment that I look so at home in my body, which is true. But to be honest, my body is still a bit more like a vacation home than it is my permanent residence. When I'm there I feel more relaxed and myself than anywhere else, but I still spend most of my life in the cramped space of my brain.

What's the difference? Well, it's the difference between what it feels like when you first sit down to practice and you can't even feel your body except to have a vague awareness (between the incessant thoughts in your head) that your chest is tight or your feet are sore—and what it feels like when you first sit up from *savasana*, a quiet buzz of aliveness in every cell and a mind that feels integrated through your whole body.

Last week I finished Matthew Sanford's book *Waking*. A paraplegic and yoga teacher, in his book Matthew tells the story of how yoga helped him bridge the distance, what he calls "the silence," between his mind and his body after trauma and years of unspeakable pain and disassociation from his body.

The book is an absolute must read. I've never known anyone to speak so beautifully and knowingly about the experience of finding oneself at home in the wholeness of one's body—physically, energetically, mentally and emotionally.

As I read it, I was of course deeply moved by the miracle of a paraplegic developing the kind of mind-body awareness Matthew has. But what I also realized, in a way that I never had before, was just how much of a miracle it is for *anyone* to have this kind of connection to his body. And thus, yet again, my appreciation for just how damned amazing yoga is deepened.

And so here's the irony—we're teaching people one of the most profound methods for staying connected to your body, and often times we're doing so from just our mind.

Why? Because we're habituated to be in our heads.

Why? Because it's really hard to be in your body!

Why?

1. Because being in your body requires practice.

Both in terms of needing to practice yoga in order to develop the capacity to be in your body and to grow your sensitivity, but also in terms of choosing to be present in your body over and over and over (and over and over) again throughout your day.

2. Because being in your body requires vulnerability.

This is in part because you can't not feel what you feel if you're present in your body. That means that aches, pains and uncomfortable or awkward emotions cannot be ignored. It also means that your lovely mind, which works so hard to keep you safe and defended and looking good, will not be the one solely in charge. And I don't know about you, but when my brain isn't the one in charge I have the same feeling as if I'm standing naked in a public place.

But on the plus side, it's being in your body that actually makes it possible for you to speak from your own experience. Because, as you may know, your own experience—the reality of it, and not the story you tell yourself and others—is in your body.

Being in your body also affords you the ability to connect with your guidance and inner knowing, so that when you're standing in front of your class with no plan, you can *feel* right there in your bones what to do next.

And finally, being in your body makes it possible for you to connect to your students more fully. When you have access to your own physical and energetic sensitivity, you can "see" other bodies more clearly, and respond to the needs of your students more expertly.

In a few words: in your body is where your life actually happens, where the present moment is felt, and thus where reality exists. And if that's true, shouldn't we all be as fierce as Matthew Sanford is about learning to stay in our body?

Going Deeper

I don't remember the moment when this thought came to me or the person I may have first heard it from, but regardless, the thought is this:

The problem with mindfulness is that it's full of mind.

Have you noticed this, too?

I can sit on my meditation cushion for hours—being mindful—and never really have a full, felt-experience of being in my body.

Similarly, I can do my entire yoga practice *mindfully*, and not at all feel connected to myself as an integrated bodymind. My mind is so persistent and strong that I can literally move through my entire day —including practicing and teaching yoga—without ever really dropping down into inhabiting my body.

So what's the difference between mindful presence and embodied presence? It's the difference between being aware that you have a body and sending your awareness *through* your body.

My friend Moira talks about mindful awareness as the experience of "being the one behind your own eyes." It's like you can watch with your awareness what is happening in your body. For example, when I'm in *trikonasana*, I can take my inner gaze down to my feet.

Embodied presence, on the other hand, is like being the one

inhabiting your whole body. It's not just looking at your feet (or heart or sacrum, etc.) in a pose with your inner gaze, it's placing your consciousness there. It happens from the inside out.

The experience of embodied presence feels soft and expansive to me, whereas mindful presence feels a bit numb and tunnel-like. The tone of it is completely different.

Just as drastic is the experience of being around someone else who is embodied versus someone who is mindful. For me, a mindful person exudes peacefulness for sure, but sometimes there is also a sense of distance or disconnection—like even though they're present, they're somehow not fully there *with me*. When I'm around a person who is really embodied, there is a palpable sense of presence. I can feel them with themselves and with me.

Take a moment right now to feel into what it feels like to you to be around someone who is really present in her body.

Take a breath.

And now take a moment to feel into being around someone who is mindful.

Which do you prefer that your students feel from you when you're teaching?

To develop a more embodied sense of presence when you teach requires that you take the time before your students show up to find yourself in your body, and to continue to do so through out all of class.

Be aware of temperature, texture, taste, sound. Notice how you feel emotionally.

Turn on your felt sense—the part of you who can feel, without looking, where the walls and windows of the room are in relationship to your body.

As your students arrive, practice staying present in your body. Continue to tune in to your felt senses as they begin to find their spots in the room.

When you begin teaching, put your own consciousness in the part of your body that you are cueing your students to work with in theirs.

Feel and hear your own breath moving as you move around the room.

When you put your hands on someone to offer an adjustment, don't lose the ability to feel your own feet on the floor.

In short, instead of having your awareness away from your body or even on your body, look for all the tiny ways you can keep your awareness in your body.

7. Don't take it all so seriously.

I have to laugh because as I sit down to write this section about not taking it all so seriously, I'm watching just how much under the surface today I've been freaking out about writing this.

I'm on the road and haven't had a chance to be near my computer much. I'm a day late in my personal deadline to finish this section, and it's nearly 6pm and I'm just starting to write. Can you sense the inner tightness and self-judgment I'm steeping in?

The reality is no one else probably gives a shit if I'm a day late in writing this section. It's just me who is going to act like the world is ending.

Kind of like how it is on those days in class when you can't for the life of you get your lefts and rights straight. Or the days when you try to articulate some kind of beautiful philosophical teaching as you direct the flow of *asana* and you end up just sounding like a wanker. Or the times when you look out into the class and can just tell that the student in the front row—the one *right* in front of you—hates what you're teaching.

Relax. It's ok. Being a yoga teacher doesn't mean you're infallible. And that's a good thing. Infallible is over-rated. And really boring.

There's juice in the mistakes. There's intimacy in the vulnerability. There's sacredness in the profane. And there's teaching in your presence, not your performance.

So don't take it all so seriously.

And yet—be serious about what you do. There is a distinction.

In my experience, taking my job as a yoga teacher too seriously means that I think I'm supposed to be something that I'm not—essentially, that I'm supposed to be perfect. It means that I hold onto negative feedback for far too long, and beat myself up over every tiny mistake. It also means that somehow the act of my yoga teaching becomes paramount in importance to all the far more consequential causes and grave events in the world.

Being serious about being a yoga teacher means that I show up with as much of me as I can, committed to my craft and open to learning. It means that I own that teaching yoga is not just a hobby and a fun thing to do, but my practice and my career. It means that I ask to be paid what I'm worth. It means that I sit with the feelings that arise when I make a mistake, but that I don't hold them over my head for all of eternity. It means that I'm dedicated to my practice, to my own personal growth and to the well-being of my students.

Going Deeper

It seems to me that if we're going to get down to the nitty gritties about not taking your teaching too seriously we need to talk about one of the main factors that causes this: our unwillingness to make mistakes or to accept them when we do.

Hard reality: You make mistakes.

Comforting reality: *Everyone* makes mistakes.

I made a royal one a few weeks ago. I mean I really screwed up. I made a commitment to a studio to come teach a workshop there, and then a few days later, once the workshop was totally full, broke my commitment because I realized I had overextended myself. If I had been checking in with myself in a deeper way when I first made the commitment I actually never would have made it. But I did, and then the only way I could be true to myself (and thus to everyone else) was to break it.

But before I wrote the lovely studio owner an email that began, "I am deeply sorry, I have made a mistake," I first spent a few days terrified of what she would say. That is to say I went through these few days as full of shame as if I had perpetrated some huge crime against humanity. I could hardly breathe from the crushing weight of my own judgment on my chest. And the commentary in my head was on par with torture techniques used on people who actually do enact crimes against humanity.

In short, I was taking the situation way too seriously. So I made a mistake. I disappointed a bunch of people and ruined a professional relationship. This kind of thing happens. As do smaller mistakes, and other fallibilities that have the potential to upset, disappoint or irritate your students, your studio owner and other teachers.

That's not to say that it's ok to continue forward unconsciously and clumsily. But do allow yourself to make mistakes and then hold yourself accountable to them when you do. I don't mean holding yourself emotionally hostage until you can somehow prove to yourself that you're a worthy human being. I mean holding yourself gently while you feel what it brings up for you that you made a mistake.

I should say this doesn't just apply to mistakes. This is about anything that makes you feel vulnerable and human in front of your students—maybe you're spent from staying up all night with your sick child, maybe you had a fight with your partner and you're distracted, maybe you'd rather be at home in bed hiding under your blankets for any number of reasons.

You don't have to have your shit together all the time. It's not possible, and it simply results in you taking yourself too seriously. You just have to be yourself and to bring your own presence to yourself to feel what you feel rather than either beating yourself up or putting on a mask. In that presence you'll find the lesson, the lightness, your humor and your humanity.

What can you do to take yourself less seriously as a teacher?

In what ways can you be more serious about your teaching?

8. Remember that your students are people.

I'm always slightly surprised by how it feels to run into a student outside of class, say, at the grocery store. There they are, wearing jeans or a suit or high heels, kids around their legs or hand-in-hand with a partner, looking for all they're worth like an honest-to-God real person.

It reminds me of what it felt like as a kid when I would run in to my schoolteacher somewhere in public. There'd be that moment of amazement when I realized that this person who I knew so intimately in the classroom actually had this whole life out in the world that I knew nothing about. I remember it feeling both unsettling (I wanted to know everything about them!), and also endearing (Oh, wow, Mrs. Hash is a mom and a wife and likes to go berry-picking, too).

Our relationship with our students can be the same way. There is an intimacy in the physicality of the practice, as well as in the emotional and spiritual inquiry, and yet there is very little dialogue. In the time that we share with our students it's mostly us talking and them listening. Not such a great model for building well-rounded relationship.

In this dynamic, it can be challenging to remember the multidimensionality of our students as people and the fact that they have a life outside of wearing yoga pants and arranging their bodies into funny shapes.

But it's not simply because we as teachers don't inquire about the lives of our students that we don't see them in their fullness; I find that people often come to yoga class as a way of escaping their life. Students walk through the studio door and want their work projects, family dynamics and all the rest of it to fall away. Students often actually willingly step into the one-dimensional role of yoga student where someone else tells them what to do.

In this way, it's incumbent upon us as yoga teachers to hold space for the multidimensionality of our students. Why? Because seeing your students one-dimensionally is a liability to teaching in a way that is truly inspiring. And because allowing your students to leave the complexity of their lives outside of the studio robs them of the full promise of their practice.

The foundation of all great teaching isn't the transmission of information, it's the relationship through which the information is shared. Your students could read about yoga in a book or watch a video, but they come to class because they want something more. They want to be in relationship. They want to be seen.

When you take the time to really see your students as people, to remember that they're carrying deadlines and heartbreaks and questions and passions in their bodies and hearts, your teaching expands. And the more you know about someone as a person, the more you care for them, and the more targeted your teaching becomes. You can access increased skill in addressing your students' needs, pushing where they need a little push, and supporting where they need a little support.

And I don't know about you, but the more students in a class who I know on a personal level, the more fun I have teaching. I find greater ease in being myself. There's a sense, no matter what we're doing in the class, that we get to hang out in and explore the thing that we have in common—being human. That's juicy. That's yoga.

Going Deeper

As I sat down to write this today and was thinking of some practical tips for how to apply remembering that your students are people, too, I came to realize just how much I *hate* it when I'm a student and I feel like all I am is a body on a mat to the person teaching.

As I was feeling into the difference between the experience of being recognized as a person versus being seen as a set of muscles and bones doing poses, I realized for the first time just how triggered I get by the latter!

Yes, perhaps I've got some personal work to do around needing to be acknowledged and seen, and yet there is no denying the importance of seeing your students as people. Teaching people yoga as opposed to teaching yoga poses is about the relationship you create with your students. Creating this relationship has to do with relating to the whole person.

With that, when it comes to remembering that your students are people, one of the simplest and greatest things you can do is to learn their names. As a student in a class, I am so much more engaged in the class and in my own process if the teacher takes the care to use my name. It's a subtle and yet significant way to remember, "Oh yeah, I'm *Jay*. Not just a body performing poses."

Not good with remembering names? That's ok. I find that *just asking* a student their name the first time they come to your class is an important gesture to let them know that you care about their individual presence in the class.

Of course, as your classes become larger it can be challenging to learn everyone's names and not possible to have time to chat with each person before or after class. This doesn't mean that there aren't more subtle ways of connecting and of making intentional room for the whole person.

One way is the difference between giving the cue "lift *the* left leg" and "lift *your* left leg." It may seem like a nit-picky difference, but it feels significantly different. When a teacher cues me in this way as a student it makes me want to scream out, "Hey, I'm in this body, you know? It's *my* foot and *my* knee, not just some random foot and knee I can direct!"

Maybe it's such a pet peeve to me as a student because I know I slip into this kind of language when I'm teaching on autopilot or checked out in some way. All in all, whether a student or a teacher, using the words "this" and "that" and "the" don't feel nearly as personal nor inspire connection nearly as much as using the words "you" and "yours."

Another big way to honor the whole person when you're teaching is to offer a number of options. The more variations you suggest for a pose, the more likely you are to meet someone where they are at physically, emotionally and energetically. This, in turn, creates a relationship between you and your student and between your student and herself rather than merely creating a picture-perfect pose.

Similar to this is teaching what the students are ready for, not what you want to teach. For example, sometimes you can come into class with an agenda to, say, teach arm balances only to find that the there are a bunch of people brand new to yoga or a person with a wrist injury or everyone is more interested in hip openers. Of course there are times when part of the teaching is facilitating your students to play up against their edges, but this is a fine art. Your job is to not just read bodies, but also to read energy and mood and to teach to who is actually in your class, not to the idea you had in your head.

There are countless other ways to remember that your students are people. If you want ideas just attend a class as a student and be curious about your experience of how the teacher interacts and talks with you.

What makes you feel seen?

What makes you feel like a piece of meat or a robot?

Given what you experience as a student, what would you do differently when you're the one leading the class?

9. Learn anatomy.

At first I hesitated to list learning anatomy as one of the 12 principles because I thought, "You know, Jay, not everyone is an anatomy geek like you are." I recognize that though some teachers like to focus on alignment, some have more of a preference for philosophy, or more interest in facilitating breath or spiritual insights. Why should they need to learn anatomy?

Before I answer that, let me digress for a moment.

As an undergraduate at the College of William and Mary, I was lucky enough to be able to take a cadaver anatomy lab. At the risk of sounding disturbed, I *loved* dissecting bodies. Being able to see with my eyes and feel with my hands things that I had only been able to know as a 2-D picture or through my inner awareness of my own body was exciting and mind-blowing.

To actually *see* what fat and connective tissue looks like, to *touch* a spinal cord, and to generally engage with the countless other amazing, mysterious, beautiful and grotesque aspects that make up the human body, absolutely and without a doubt changed the way that I inhabit my body. It also changed the way that I practice and teach yoga.

I remember that I would leave anatomy lab to go straight to

practice with my teacher, and I'd be sitting in *janu sirsasana* and I'd want to be able to run my finger down the length of the belly of my medial hamstring like I had done with the cadaver earlier in the day.

Well not really—the whole part about cutting through my skin first and pain receptors and all that definitely ruled out any benefit of how good it would have felt to have the muscle smoothed out. But the thing was, knowing what it felt like to run my finger down the belly of a hamstring affected my felt experience of my hamstring in the pose. It also influenced how I read and understood the bodies of my students in forward folds.

Before I continue telling more gruesome stories (which I love to do because I'm the daughter and granddaughter of nurses), let me come back to the question of why yoga teachers should learn anatomy.

Well, frankly, because I think *everybody* should learn anatomy. Every body. I know that sounds soap boxy, but I just think that since every single one of us spends every single second of our life in one of these miraculous things called a human body, that we would want to actually know what they look like on the inside and maybe a bit about how they work.

Even if you never apply it in any formal way. For example, I have no intention of becoming a mechanic, but I drive a car all the time and I think it's interesting to at least pop open the hood and see what the engine looks like. And I've found it quite useful to know how to change my own oil and change a flat tire.

But that's the thing: yoga teachers actually *do* apply anatomy every time they teach, even if you don't ever use the name of a specific bone or muscle or mention its action or function.

The body is our medium the way clay is for a sculptor or food is for a chef. This seems obvious when you're teaching *asana* or even *pranayama*, but even if your main focus is on teaching the *sutras*, anatomy still applies because, as humans, we experience everything through the felt experience and intelligence of our body. Knowing more about the body helps you to teach the whole person and not just convey a pose or an idea.

Our bodies are a huge part of what makes us similar. There are really only variations on two themes—male and female. And yet, there are so many variations! No two cadavers that I got to work on had anything the same—muscle size, joint functioning, organ health —just the same way that each of your students have unique variations, as well.

The more you know about anatomy, the more you can meet the physical needs of your students, which means you have more aptitude for meeting the mental, emotional and spiritual needs, too.

Going Deeper

Over the years of talking with hundreds of yoga teachers I have never met a teacher who wasn't supremely grateful for having received extensive training in anatomy. Unfortunately, this is a small group of people.

Similarly, I can't recall ever meeting a single teacher who has said that he feels like he doesn't need to or care to know anything more about anatomy. We as yoga teachers can all humbly admit that having a limited understanding of muscle functioning and location, joint articulation, fascial restrictions and any number of other anatomical workings limits our ability to address the needs of our students.

In this way, learning anatomy is one of the most important principles for teaching a person instead of teaching a pose. The ability to understand the unique body of each student allows you to work with that student in a more personal way.

And yet, it's important to point out that knowing anatomy in a scholarly way is far different than knowing anatomy in an experiential way. Cueing a student to internally rotate this, abduct that, or supinate this has absolutely no benefit unless you can feel in your own body what that means and articulate why someone would want to do that.

In fact, relying on a heady understanding of "correct alignment" leads to a tendency to encourage students to fix rather than feel their poses, and to favor precision at the expense of intuition. This in turn reduces the whole operation to the performance of a pose rather than to facilitating a person finding her own inner alignment.

By inner alignment I don't mean a body free of discomfort or the best pose that a person can do. Though these things will be inherent side effects of inner alignment, what I mean is that the person has a sense on all levels of being *aligned with himself*. A feeling of being at ease, present and fully alive.

Though I highly recommend learning as much as you can about applied anatomy through books and courses (especially those specific to the anatomy of yoga), I cannot stress enough the importance of studying your own experience in the poses. There is such a vast amount of information available on the inside of one's experience. And yet, so many people never tap into this inner wisdom because it takes so much sensitivity, energy and attention to access it.

In fact, in comparison to becoming masterful at being able to track the movement of breath, to sense the slightest shift in physical sensation, or to ride the continuous waves of emotional fluctuations, having to memorize hundreds of muscles and their attachment and insertion points seems a hell of a lot less daunting.

But the good news is, one acts in service of the other: Felt experience serves anatomical knowledge and anatomical knowledge serves felt experience.

For example, when I was studying anatomy in college, I marveled at how I essentially got to have a cheat sheet with me at every test; here were all these questions about the human body, and I happened to be sitting there in a human body! Not that I could necessarily see all the structures that I was asked about, but I could *feel* them. I could stand up right there in the aisle of desks and check it out for myself, "What *does* the quadratus lumborum do if I flex it?"

Similarly, after years of studying *Iyengar* yoga in which there was a continuous onslaught of external alignment cues to follow, I found myself interested in styles of yoga that were more internal, introspective and subtle. What I discovered was that when I could slow down and listen attentively to how my body wanted to move in order to feel easeful and open, I could *feel* my way into the pose from the inside out. The movements weren't any different than what my *Iyengar* teacher had verbally cued me on, they simply came from my body's intelligence.

With that, trust that you have all the information you need about movement and alignment in your own body, it just requires that you pay attention. Take the time to feel what you're doing when you practice. Sense what happens so that the anatomical cues make sense to you.

Buy an anatomy of yoga book. Rather than just studying the pictures, pick one pose each practice and actually play with sensing what muscles are working and how in the pose.

When you go to a class as a student, experiment with the cues your teacher offers. What happens if you externally rotate your shoulder like she suggests? What happens if you don't?

When you're practicing at home on your own, talk to yourself out loud about what you're doing and how it feels. Use what you discover through your own experience to craft cues that you can offer your students.

10. Plan enough so that you can be spontaneous.

Years ago my dad jokingly asked me what would happen if I ever lost my trusty Moleskine day planner. I shuddered to think.

I *love* me a plan.

I love mapping out my days, weeks and months in great detail. Not only in said planner, but also constantly in my mind. I love walking into the yoga studio with the safety blanket of a cleverly crafted sequence in my back pocket. I even (and I hate admitting it) have the tendency to plan out the trajectory of an entire relationship during the first date. As you can see, it's a bit of a problem.

But I'm getting much better at letting go of my plan out in the world, in the studio and in relationships. Why? Because I'm finally coming to accept the fact that having a plan just doesn't work.

And not only that, but I'm coming to see that it's a good thing that having a plan doesn't work because it means that I'm actually more connected to what's really happening in the moment as opposed to my limited idea of what would be best.

There's a line from a David Whyte poem that I absolutely love that speaks to this: *"What you can plan is too small for you to live."*

What this means to me is that each moment, each interaction, each idea is big and pregnant with possibility and aliveness. If we come to it with the restrictive energy of a plan we're not making space for the magic and learning that could have been birthed through real-time relating to and living of that moment.

Feel into it for yourself. You know what it feels like to come into the studio with the whole hour and a half mapped out and to stick to your plan even if it doesn't quite fit the situation. For example, you've planned out a killer sequence of deep backbends only to come to a class full of relatively new students and a couple of folks with minor back injuries.

If you stick to your plan you will be operating on autopilot in disconnection from your students. You might be going through the motions of a teacher who can put together a kick ass sequence, but who really cares if it doesn't actually serve the people who are there?

In fact, it shows little regard for the people who are there because you have to stay partially (if not a lot) shut down or disassociated to their experience in order to stay in allegiance with your plan. Not good.

The other end of the spectrum is not having a plan whatsoever. Having absolutely no stinking clue of anything you want to do, say or invoke. This *can* work, but only if you are incredibly present, on your game, willing to be vulnerable, and have a good amount of resources in terms of your knowledge of the practice of yoga. When this works, nothing can beat it—these are the classes that feel the most connected and blissful and mindboggingly synchronistic.

But when it doesn't work, it can lead to where I was last week when I taught without a plan, without having had a long enough self-practice to actually get clear and present, in a new space with all new students: the yoga teacher equivalent of a fish flailing around on the shore, gasping for air. Not pretty.

So that's why it's good to plan enough to allow for spontaneity. One of my mentors from rites of passage work calls this creating enough form to allow for freedom. You'll know when you've found the right balance because you'll feel confident, grounded, open and creative.

Going Deeper

We've all been there. You plan the most intelligent series of hip openers and then everyone in class requests shoulder work. You have a beautiful *dharma* talk on non-violence planned only to realize that the topic of the day on your students' hearts is fear. You plan to have a cozy restorative class only to find that the heat in the studio is broken.

The gist: the universe almost always laughs at your plans.

And yet, having *some* idea of what you want to teach is useful.

So the questions become *Why do you plan?* And How much do you *really need to plan?*

Why do you plan?

I'm aware of 3 reasons that I plan:

1. Because I have a specific skill or technique or concept that I want my students to learn. For example, if I have set a theme of inversion for my classes for a month, I'll plan a series of classes that are preparatory for inversions, sequentially and skillfully getting closer and closer to actually going upside down.

2. Because I feel shut down or not centered for some reason and I need something to hold onto. The plan becomes a security blanket so that I have something to teach when I can't actually feel what's

present in the moment. For sure, this is not ideal, but sometimes it's the best I can do.

3. Similar to #2, when I first started teaching I planned *every moment* of a class. Everything about teaching was demanding and sometimes overwhelming and I needed to feel like I wasn't totally drowning! The more comfortable I've become as a teacher and the more familiar I've become with the practice of yoga in general, the less I need to plan.

Which leads me to ask...How much do you really need to plan?

This, of course, depends on the individual and on the type of yoga you teach. But akin to what I was saying in #3 above, the more familiar you are with the practice and with teaching, the easier it is to have less of a plan.

I notice on days that I have had a long or particularly insightful self-practice I need less of a plan when I go to teach. My body and my intuition are sensitive enough in the moment to sense not only what's needed, but also how to respond from my own experience and expertise.

And though it's true that the longer I've been teaching, the more comfortable I feel with playing in the moment with what works in terms of sequencing, *dharma* themes, etc., I recognize that this is only true precisely because I spent years meticulously planning and having studied (both in a scholarly way as well as in an experientially way) poses that have similar anatomical considerations and emotional and psychological themes.

I can't stress enough how useful it has been for me to build an inner library of hip openers, external shoulder openers, poses that are calming or inspiring or fierce, etc. My recommendation to you is that if you don't have a strong sense of thematic grouping and interrelation of poses, start making lists now. Practice the poses with the question in mind—what are the anatomical considerations and spiritual/emotional/psychological themes that this pose embodies?

Also, feel for overlaps in poses that have similar considerations that might go well together in a sequence. That way when you show up to teach class and someone asks for heart opening and another person for hamstring stretches you can go in to the Venn Diagram in your brain and pull out the handful of poses that address both of those things at once.

Once you have this body of knowledge to pull from, you can play with how much you plan. Some days you might still plan the whole shebang—every pose in the sequence, the philosophical or spiritual theme or question, maybe even a reading. Other days maybe it's just one pose you really want to do, or perhaps a poem you'd like to share. Then you get to class and see how what you have to share weaves in to what you feel is needed.

All that said, the most general answer to the question of how much do you need to plan is this: Plan enough that you can really be of service to your students. Some days this will be more of a plan, some days less. But being of service to your students' safety, growth and insight is what the plan (or lack thereof) is all about.

What do you need to plan?

How can you make a class structure that allows for enough breathing room to honor who and what shows up once you get to the studio?

What are you willing to let go of the moment you walk into the studio? Or twenty minutes into class?

How can you be more permeable and available to the present situation as you teach?

What do you notice happens when you allow for more spontaneity in your teaching?

11. Remember who and what supports you.

I think it's pretty safe to say that most yoga teachers are caretakers. We have an inherent gift for offering care and attention and for supporting others in their process. This is wonderful, and it's a major reason why we're good at what we do.

And yet, I've also recognized that we're not so good at receiving support. And this limitation is one thing that keeps us from being truly remarkable at what we do.

I know I can get into the mindset when I go into the studio to teach that the growth and general well-being of everyone in the room rests on my shoulders. I know, it sounds crazy and conceited, but it's unconscious—and I think fairly common among card-carrying caretakers.

The reality is: The magic that happens in a class happens because you show up as fully as you can. And that's only one piece. The other equally as important piece is that you also get out of your own way as much as you can. Both need to happen.

What do I mean by get out of your own way? I mean remember who and what supports you—and *let it* support you. Even though it can feel like you're standing up there in front of your class totally alone, that just ain't the case. Ever.

So what kind of support?

Well, to begin with, there's the ground. Ridiculously obvious, I know. But how often are you actually consciously aware of the ground underneath you when you teach? Believe me, it makes a difference when you are. And the brilliant thing about the ground is that it's always there. You just have to become aware of it in order to feel more grounded.

On a different part of the tangibility spectrum is the collective field. Way cool research about physics, the Tao and collective consciousness is out there now that talks about how when a group of people come together for a specific purpose there is an underlying pattern of intelligence in their collective energetic field. (This is one of my favorite geeky subjects.)

It sounds kind of out there when you try to talk about it, but you've probably experienced it. It's that thing that happens when you find yourself talking about some seemingly random topic during your class only to have a student come up to you afterward and tell you that that very thing just happened to them.

Somehow you've tapped into an intelligence or shared consciousness that is in the room. This is quite possibly one of the most exciting experiences of teaching. A bit harder than letting the ground beneath you support you, but no less real if you can be present enough to tap into the insights and gut feelings that seem to come out of nowhere as you teach.

And then there's your personal relationship to what you understand as Spirit, or the grace that exists in all things. How do you relate to that as you teach? I personally always start class by lighting a candle and silently inviting Spirit to be present with me so that I can feel it's presence in the room, in my students, and in myself in the form of my own guidance when I teach. Every time my eyes glance by the candle it's a reminder to me to relax and to let myself feel more supported by that which I can't see.

These are just a few of my sources of support, but I know that there are many, many different kinds. What or who are *your* sources of support? How do you acknowledge them? How could you rest into them more in the moments when you are teaching?

One last thing. This is where I'd like to mention the importance of having a teacher, a counselor and some network of support of other professionals. I can't stress this enough. If you're going to support others in exploring their edges, you need to have someone who supports you in that. If you're going to encourage your students to deepen their practice, you have to have someone do that for you. Do you have a teacher? A mentor? A counselor? A spiritual director?

A circle of colleagues you meet with?

Not only will having this kind of support make your life feel far more sane, it's what helps you to see and to learn from your own experience so that you can help others to do the same. And it's kind of not a choice: *You need this kind of support*. Believe me. I taught for years without any immediate outside support, and it was no bueno. Why? Because having other people who call you up and call you out is a major factor in your integrity as a person and as a teacher. So find some support!

Going Deeper

I was reminded this afternoon of a memory from childhood that I hadn't thought of in some time. I was an elite level gymnast as a kid, and at some point in my young career I developed a mental block to back flips on the balance beam.

Even though it was something my body was completely capable of doing, my mind would take over and say that I couldn't. Not only that I couldn't, but that if I did, very, very bad things would happen, like concussions and broken necks.

And so I would stand there, absolutely frozen. Minute, after minute, after minute.

I would start by endeavoring to give myself a countdown (5, 4, 3, 2, 1, GO!) because if I didn't think about it, my body would just do the trick. Then I could go on with the rest of my routine.

But this didn't always work. My fear would be too great to get centered, and I would need something more. So I would ask my coach to stand closer. She didn't have to touch me, or even have her arm raised toward me. I just wanted her closer. I wanted to feel her eyes on me, her presence with me.

And then some days, especially when adding difficulty to a trick, I knew I needed my coach's hand right there on my lower back. And maybe even some extra crash pads.

So as I write about remembering *who* and *what* supports you in your teaching, it dawns on me that part of this inquiry is also being clear with *when* and *how* you need support, too.

Because, well, support can be tricky. Some of us don't have nearly enough support in terms of not having a teacher or a counselor or a way of grounding in the moments of our teaching. Some of us rely too heavily on the spots and the crash pads.

The thing to remember with support is that true support always brings you back to your *own* sense of agency and confidence, not your need to rely on something or someone outside of you. A person who offers you support with integrity does so in a way that makes space for your fear and insecurities and doubts, whether rational or not, but does not enable them.

As you consider your sources of support, which ones bring you back to your own center? Which ones feel like crutches?

Are you aware of where you could use more support? Or perhaps where you're ready to rely upon less external support?

12. Don't try to please everyone.

Don't try to please everyone. Because you can't.

(And, God, how my fragile little ego wishes it weren't true!)

I mean, I get that trying to please everyone is a recipe for disaster, and that it's actually *not even possible* to please everyone, and yet it wasn't (let me be honest here: *isn't*) an easy thing for me to actually learn how to apply in practice.

I first started teaching yoga when I was 18 and I wasn't yet down with my vulnerability or my expertise. All I was really clear on was that I desperately wanted my students to like me.

So every time a student gave me feedback after class, I would jump to accommodate them in the next class. More sun salutations? Ok. Less talking? Yes, ma'am! Arrange the room differently. You betcha.'

I got to the point where each class that I showed up to teach was a whole new me and a completely different kind of class. This had the effect of me feeling constantly lost when I was teaching. And of course, because of this, I kept getting more and more feedback as to how I could make my class "better."

And so this is how the twelfth principle brings us full circle back to the first, be yourself.

Because:

Truth: The very act of being yourself will sometimes disappoint, hurt, frustrate and repel other people (which you will almost always be painfully aware of).

Truth: *Not* being yourself will *always* disappoint, hurt, frustrate and repel yourself (which is harder to be sensitive to at first, but far more painful and destructive).

The reality is the reason you try to please everyone is so that you won't have to feel un-liked or alone. And yet, it's inevitable—not everyone is going to like you and, in a way, you're kind of always alone in your own experience.

So the important questions are: Can *you* like you? Can you not abandon yourself?

This is big. And this isn't just about teaching yoga, but about being a human being. Can you get to the point where your allegiance to yourself becomes more important than pleasing someone else?

In your teaching, this is the place where you become brilliant— when you stop worrying what other people will think. Or maybe you still worry, and get hurt when you disappoint someone, but you have the resources, both inner and outer, to support yourself in doing the work you need to do in order to continue being more and more yourself.

And you can comfort yourself in all of this by saying, "some people may not like me, and they'll stop coming to my classes, but I'll attract the people who do like me and they will stay."

But be careful about putting too much stock in this, because I would also say this: unless some of your students don't like you some of the time you're not being as brilliant a teacher as you are capable of.

How do I know this? Because *my* favorite teachers are the ones who I respect and trust—and whom I also don't always like. That's because they challenge who and how I am, which tweaks me out and makes me project all my stuff on them and hate them. Sometimes. And then when I break through to a different level of embodied understanding because of their teaching, I realize just how much I love them and am grateful for their willingness to not be liked by me.

Get it? To be an inspirational teacher with integrity, your students need you to do your work so that you can be ok with not pleasing people all of the time. It's both liberating and terrifying.

But it really isn't about what your students need. In fact, none of the 12 Principles are really only about that. They're about you getting to be you in the world—no matter what you're doing—in the most alive, connected and real way.

Going Deeper

The early years of my teaching were plagued with worrying about trying to please everyone in class. These were not my most successful years as a teacher. I wasn't clear with who I was as a teacher and what it was that was true for me to teach, and I was hooked on external approval. Because of this, I got a *lot* of feedback from my students about how I could improve.

About seven years in to my teaching, I was less hooked on making sure everyone in the room was happy, and a little more clear about my own style of teaching, but I still got quite a bit of feedback. Students would come up to me after class and let me know what worked for them and what didn't, and how they thought the class could be better.

At this point, I was able to see that, other than a handful of really helpful suggestions, what my students shared with me was mostly *their* stuff (preferences, triggers, projections), and that I couldn't possibly try to accommodate everyone's feedback (nor would it be useful for anyone if I tried).

I was proud of myself when, after weeks on end of telling me why my class was not what she wanted, I looked the opinionated student right in the eye and cleanly said, "This is how I teach. Here is my boss's contact information—please contact her and tell her why you think they should take this class away from me, and if you're not alone in holding that opinion, I will happily leave. Until then, either choose to attend or to not attend class, but I no longer want your feedback."

Interestingly, that woman continued to come to class. Not only that, she stopped telling me how to teach my class and started participating with what I was offering.

On the opposite end of the spectrum from the students who offer their opinion about every small thing you do (and far more common), are the students who never say anything. You read their expressions and body language to get a sense for how they respond to your teaching. But for the most part, you can only guess at what's going on with your students in terms of why they like your teaching or not, what games they're playing or not, what they want and don't want. And putting energy into figuring out what your students want only creates more controlling or confused students and a more spun-out you.

Because here's what I notice: I don't get this kind of feedback now after my classes, the kind where a student tells me how they think I could change or tweak something to make my class a better fit for what they need and want. I still get questions and insights and suggestions for something I might want to research, but not suggestions on how to teach. And I still see where someone may not enjoy my class, but they don't feel compelled to tell me about it. They simply just don't return.

So what's changed?

I've changed. I'm more certain in what I have to offer—even on my worst days, I'm more comfortable in my skin as a teacher and more clear and purposeful about how I teach. I don't send out an energetic plea for help and feedback—I share what I have to share in an embodied and confident way. In my clarity, my students get to feel if what I have to offer resonates or not, and choose accordingly.

I'm not suggesting that receiving feedback, solicited or not, is in any way bad or suggests that you're not clear in your teaching. Quite the contrary! It's important to get feedback, and an art to truly receive it—sometimes *especially* as you're more comfortable with your teaching style.

I'm just suggesting that you consider how much and what kind of feedback you're getting. If you're getting a lot of the variety about how you could change this or change that to make the class experience better for your students, you might want to pause and ask your inner wise self:

Is this feedback true—would it really serve everyone involved if I did what they asked?

If not, ask yourself if you're clear with what it is you want to offer or if you're valuing your students' happiness and good opinion over your own truth?

Conclusion

When I first wrote the 12 Principles, I called them "tips for transformational teaching." In the final stages of editing this book I dropped the term "transformational" because the word implies that something needs to be different, needs to change in order for you or your students to be better, more evolved or somehow more acceptable.

The truth is, even after writing the 12 Principles from my own lived experience, I still got lured in by the sex appeal of the word "transformational." The desire to be different, to morph into a new and improved version of the self, is just so deeply ingrained.

Though, yes, you will change and grow—as will your students— when you employ the 12 Principles of *Teaching People, Not Poses*, neither the intent behind them nor the outcome of their practice is transformation.

When it comes down to it, *Teaching People, Not Poses* is about having *integrity*. Integrity in the sense of being more whole. More yourself. Bringing together all the parts of you, and not hiding or holding back.

But also integrity in terms of alignment. In this case, alignment with your truth, as opposed to contorting yourself to fit what other people expect of you.

Though there is a lot of lip service given to pursuing your whole and truthful self, especially in the yoga community, the reality is that it remains unpopular in practice. The underlying message seems to be, " Be your whole and truthful self—as long as it falls within the acceptable bandwidth of being loving, compassionate and spiritual.

And while you're at it, get a sweaty workout to ensure you can be as physically beautiful as you can." In this way, there is an awful lot of posing and posturing in yoga.

That's not to dump on being loving, compassionate and spiritual. That's wonderful—when that's what's true for you. But what about when it's not? Where's your place in yoga when you're feeling hateful, annoyed and full of doubt?

Similarly, there's nothing inherently horrible about yoga being a good workout. In fact, it's great! Our bodies need exercise, and yoga is one of the most intelligent ways to do so. But simply relegating yoga to the category of "a good workout" robs it of its stunning complexity.

Yoga offers so much more than this surface-level posturing towards some theoretical ideal of physical and spiritual "perfection." In this way, despite (or because of) its mainstream popularity, yoga is not living up to it's potential. So what unlocks yoga's true potential as a vast and complex system of support for realizing the Self and the self?

You do.

Who you are as a teacher and what you bring to your teaching is one of *the* deciding factors for the direction that yoga will take in our culture. How you teach influences your students' focus on their mat, and thus what they take with them into their lives and into their communities.

Yes, most people go to yoga these days because they want a workout. And yes, teaching a workout is a hell of a lot easier than facilitating being and becoming. So why not play the role of yoga guru? Why not let your students go into autopilot while you direct their every peaceful breath and sweaty move?

Because I think the majority of people want a workout from their yoga simply because they don't know any better. Like their tight hamstring muscles and sore lower backs from too much sitting, it's just what they've gotten used to. It's habituated. It's affirmed by social norms.

Or maybe they know yoga can be much more than a workout, but keeping the practice purely physical keeps it safe. Orienting toward the performance of a pose—whether as a teacher or as a student— keeps yoga about external forms of measurement and superficial change. Again, things that we're used to.

But just as I refuse to believe that people are truly ok with living with chronic back pain, I also refuse to believe that people are ok with moving through their lives without true connection, without risking following the quiet yet persistent voice of their own deepest self, without a felt sense of their own tender and indestructible spirit.

And yet, it's one of the most challenging things in the world to let go of numbness and tightness and truly stretch and open ourselves to our own sensitivity and strength. In essence, to be ourselves.

It's hard because it's scary as hell and because we lack role models in how to do this.

And we lack role models in how to do this because it's hard and scary as hell.

That's where teaching yoga with integrity comes in.

If you're willing as a teacher to go to the places that scare you, to soften when you want to get hard and to attend to the complexity of your life through your practice, your students will also learn to do so. And that means more people in your community and in our world who dare to live in integrity. And that, my friends, we need for oh so many reasons.

I know it's hard. I know it's scary. But it's worth it. Because at the end of the day, *Teaching People, Not Poses* isn't really only about teaching yoga. It's about playing your part to help create a world full of people who have the courage and the spirit to set aside fear and to live in alignment with their deepest, truest most full self.

It happens one person at a time. And it starts with you. You as you are right now, no transformation necessary.

Shine.

Acknowledgements

I would like to honor some specific people in my lineage and community who have greatly influenced me, my learning and the publication of this book.

Rosie Taylor for setting such a solid foundation for yoga in my body, heart, mind and spirit. Who knew I'd still be teaching all these years later?

Cinda Friedman and Julie Gudmestad for continually facilitating me back to my own soft, strong center with fierce compassion and expertise from your own practices.

My dear friend Mandy Blake for always being there for sanity checks, last-minute edits, geeky chats, celebrations and so much more.

Moira McNairnay for being a muse, a fellow "player" and a friend.

Cheryl Ramette, Sasha Davies and Michelle Hynes for the alchemy of our collective learning and living.

The Nooners for creating a teaching atmosphere in which I finally found *me*.

And as always, my family, for among many things, believing in me.

About the Author

Jay Fields, M.A. RYT believes in the power of yoga to help people to connect to their humanity as well as to their divinity. Having taught yoga since 1998 and having earned a master's degree in Integral Transformative Education, she doesn't just teach poses, she teaches the whole person.

Jay teaches classes and leads workshops for teachers and students nationally and internationally, and mentors yoga teachers in how to be more human when they teach. For more information on Jay's teaching and writing, please visit www.jay-fields.com.

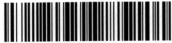